AMAZING BODY RESET PLAN:

Bringing your body to a perfect balanced state

Ruth D.Palafox

Table of contents

This challenge is meant to help you reset your system for improved energy, deeper sleep, stress alleviation and to nurture your relationship with food. So what do you need to do for greater sleep and vitality in only one fortnight?

I will counsel you to cut out alcohol and urge you to explore vitamin-rich meals to be for ingestion.

During the body reset challenge, it's vital to prepare nutritious meals to consume throughout the week and integrate energy-rich foods into your diet.

This challenge is meant to help you reset your system for improved energy, deeper sleep, stress alleviation and to nurture your relationship with food.

During the two-week reset challenge, it's crucial to prepare nutritious meals to consume throughout the week and integrate energy-rich foods into your diet

FOODS TO EAT MORE OF DURING THE RESET:

Greens - at every meal

Gluten-free grains — brown rice, gluten-free oats, quinoa, and buckwheat

White fish and salmon - 2-3 times a week

Organic chicken and eggs

Legumes - e.g. beans, lentils, and chickpeas

Fruits - berries, lemon, green apples, grapefruit, papaya

Root veggies - potato, sweet potato, pumpkin, beetroot, parsnip

Nut milk

Oils – extra virgin olive oil

All herbs and spices

Wholesome condiments - lemon juice, Dijon mustard, tahini, tamari

Consume less caffeine, sugar and no alcohol should be ingested, caffeine should be confined to just one cup per day before 11 am.

While this may seem like a struggle in itself, the physical advantages are tremendously useful for general health and well-being.

As a coffee alternative, I would suggest you consume spicy turmeric latte or dandelion root tea, as both are pleasant and flavourful.

Refined sugar, artificial sweeteners, soft drinks, and soda should also be minimized.

Alcohol should not be used and caffeine should be confined to one cup per day throughout the weeklong reset

FOOD AND DRINK TO REDUCE:

Caffeine - restricted to one cup of coffee each day before 11 am

Alcohol - during the length of the challenge

Refined sugar and artificial sweeteners

Red meat - strive for organic and grass-fed

Soda and soft drinks

Gluten and dairy - if sensitive

Hydrate your body

As the human body comprises about 60 percent water, it is necessary to preserve health and well-being by drinking at least two liters of water each day.

I would also advocate drinking up to 2.5L of water every day as well as drinking herbal teas and coconut water if feasible.

Adequate consumption of water can help hydrate the kidneys, enhance digestion and intestinal health, rejuvenate the skin and prevent feeling weary.

We lose a lot of water through consuming caffeinated beverages, such as teas and coffees, and overnight when sleeping - therefore we need to replace this during the day.

On top of eating correctly, it's encouraged to exercise at least once a day, but those ready for an additional challenge may train twice every day.

The idea is to practice at least 20 minutes of 'targeted exercise' every day to enjoy the health and mental advantages.

Depending on your chosen form of training, cardio or weights may be mixed into each exercise to challenge the body in various ways - as cardio can assist burn fat, while weights aid grow muscle.

Chapter 1

Possible causes of belly fat

Getting rid of extra belly fat, or abdominal fat is a typical aim for many.

While keeping a reasonable body weight and body fat percentage is vital for overall health, the sort of belly fat you accumulate might affect your health differently.

The two primary kinds are:

visceral\ssubcutaneous

Visceral refers to fat around the liver and other abdominal organs. Having large amounts of visceral fat is related to an elevated risk for chronic illnesses such as metabolic syndrome, type 2 diabetes, heart disease, and some forms of cancer.

On the other hand, subcutaneous is the layer of fat that resides right beneath the skin. This form is less detrimental to health and acts as a layer of protection for your organs as well as insulation to regulate body temperature.

That said, having a large level of subcutaneous fat is related to a bigger amount of visceral fat, hence raising your risk of health issues.

Focusing on a health-promoting lifestyle, which helps avoid excessive levels of both kinds of fat, is vital

Here are 11 variables that might contribute to the development of extra abdominal fat:

1. Sugary meals and drinks; Many individuals eat more added sugar every day than they think.

Common items in the diet that might be rich in added sugar include baked goods, pastries, muffins, flavored yogurts, morning cereals, granola and protein bars, prepackaged meals, and sugar-sweetened drinks (SSBs), and other processed foods.

In particular, a diet heavy in SSBs (e.g., sodas, specialty coffees, fruit juices, energy drinks) is related to increased visceral abdominal fat SSBs are the major source of sugar intake owing to their cheap cost, convenience, and simplicity of ingestion. Unlike food, SSBs may be ingested fast in large amounts because they need minimum preparation.

As a consequence, you experience a massive intake of calories and sugar, with little to no nutritious benefit, in a single sitting. For many, it's not unusual to eat numerous SSBs in a single day.

For example, consuming two 16 fluid ounce (480 mL) bottles of soda in a day adds up to 384 calories and 104 grams of sugar. This, particularly if taken in addition to many other high-sugar meals and beverages, may contribute to excessive calorie consumption in a day and, eventually, excess visceral fat.

Furthermore, drinking your calories – especially from SSBs – may lead to a transient boost in blood sugar followed by a collapse, leading to you feeling hungry rapidly and having to drink or eat soon again.

Though some argue the high-fructose corn syrup (HFCS) in SSBs is the major contributor to visceral fat, most evidence shows that HFCS and ordinary sugar (sucrose) both contribute to weight gain similarly – i.e., by delivering excessive calories – rather than having a distinct role in fat storage.

While all meals and drinks may be enjoyed in moderation, it's preferable to restrict sugar-sweetened food and beverages to special occasions. Instead, choose water, unsweetened coffee/tea, and unprocessed, less processed meals most frequently. A diet heavy in added sugars, particularly sugar-sweetened drinks, may increase belly fat. Most typically, stay with water, unsweetened coffee/tea, and eating a diet rich in whole, minimally processed foods.

2. Alcohol

Alcohol may have both beneficial and detrimental consequences. When ingested at modest levels, particularly as red wine, it is connected with decreased risk of heart disease.

However, heavy alcohol consumption may lead to inflammation, liver disease, some forms of cancer, excess weight gain, and many other health concerns.

Therefore, the Centers for Disease Control and Prevention (CDC) suggest no more than one drink per day for women and two drinks per day for men or avoiding alcohol.

Additionally, heavy alcohol use is connected with increased visceral fat buildup and a higher body mass index.

It's claimed that alcohol leads to belly fat and general weight increase in a few ways

Alcohol has a large number of calories (7 calories per gram) (7 calories per gram).

Many alcoholic drinks are rich in sugar.

Alcohol may stimulate hunger and lower inhibitions, leading to increased total calorie consumption.

Alcohol may lead to worse judgment, leading to higher eating of less nutritious meals.

It may change hormones associated with appetite and fullness.

It may inhibit fat oxidation, which may save stored fat. Though further study is required.

It may elevate cortisol, which increases belly fat accumulation.

A person may be less eager to be physically active the day before and after drinking.

Alcohol contributes to worse sleep quality, which is related to increased BMI and fat accumulation.

A comprehensive evaluation of 127 research indicated a strong dose-dependent connection between alcohol intake and belly fat accumulation.

Other studies have shown demonstrated a high alcohol consumption (2–3 drinks or more per day) is connected to weight increase including abdominal obesity, particularly in males.

If you prefer to drink, aim for no more than 1–2 drinks each day.

High alcohol intake (more than two drinks per day) is connected with weight growth and abdominal fat.

3. Trans fats.

Trans fats are among the unhealthiest fats.

While minor quantities of trans fat exist in nature, they're typically manufactured for the food system by adding hydrogen to unsaturated fats to make them more stable and enable them to be solid at room temperature.

Trans fats are widely utilized in baked goods and packaged meals as a cheap — but effective — alternative for butter, lard, and higher-cost commodities.

Artificial trans fats have been demonstrated to promote inflammation, which may lead to insulin resistance, heart disease, some forms of cancer, and several other disorders. However, ruminant trans fats, which are present naturally in dairy and meat products, do not have the same harmful health consequences.

Though it's suspected that trans fat may also lead to visceral fat — and has been related to bad health over previous decades — there's a little contemporary study on the matter.

Even with many nations having taken efforts to restrict or prohibit the use of artificial trans fats in the food supply, it's crucial to still read the nutrition label if you're uncertain.

Artificial trans fats are closely related to poor heart health and may also contribute to increased belly fat. Both the US and Canada have prohibited trans fats in commercial foods.

4. Sedentary lifestyle and physical inactivity

A sedentary lifestyle is one of the largest risk factors for bad health occurrences. It includes extended sitting throughout the day (e.g., watching TV, sitting at a work desk, lengthy commuting, playing video games, etc). (e.g., watching TV, sitting at a work desk, long commutes, playing video games, etc.).

Even if a person is physically active, meaning they engage in physical labor or exercise, prolonged sitting may increase the risk of negative health events and weight gain.

Additionally, data reveals that the majority of children and adults do not reach the recommended physical activity standards.

To further underline the harmful impact limiting exercise has on the body, both physical inactivity and a sedentary lifestyle have been related to a direct rise in both visceral and subcutaneous belly fat. Fortunately, participating in regular physical exercise and reducing sitting throughout the day may minimize your risk of increasing belly fat while supporting weight control.

In one study, researchers discovered that persons who undertook resistance or aerobic exercise for 1 year after losing weight were able to avoid regaining visceral fat, but those who did not exercise had a 25–38 percent rise in belly fat.

Another research found that individuals who sat for over 8 hours each day (not counting sleeping hours) had a 62 percent greater risk of obesity compared with those who sat for less than 4 hours each day.

It's advised that most individuals strive for at least 150 minutes of moderate aerobic physical exercise (or 75 minutes of strenuous activity) per week and participate in regular resistance training.

Further, aim to reduce sedentary activities and extended sitting. If sitting is part of your job, try to integrate "standing breaks" every 30–90 minutes by standing for 5–10 minutes or taking a brisk stroll around your workplace, house or neighborhood.

A sedentary lifestyle and physical inactivity are related to a multitude of health hazards, including weight gain and increased belly fat. Aim for at least 150 minutes of moderate to intense physical exercise per week.

5. Low protein diet

Consuming enough dietary protein may promote weight control.

High protein diets may assist weight reduction and prevent weight gain by increasing fullness, because protein takes longer to digest compared to other macronutrients. Protein also helps muscle repair and development, which adds to a greater metabolism and more calories expended at rest.

Several studies reveal that persons who eat the largest quantity of protein are the least likely to develop extra abdominal fat.

To improve your protein consumption, strive to incorporate a high quality protein source at each meal and snack, such as lean meat, chicken, tofu, eggs, beans, and lentils. High protein consumption is connected with decreased belly fat and moderate body weight.

6. Menopause

Gaining belly fat after menopause is quite frequent.

At puberty, the hormone estrogen tells the body to begin accumulating fat on the hips and thighs in preparation for a prospective pregnancy. This subcutaneous fat isn't dangerous from a health aspect, but it may be tough to remove in certain situations.

Menopause officially occurs one year after a woman experiences her last menstrual cycle. Around this period, estrogen levels decline considerably. Though menopause affects individual woman differently, in general it tends to cause fat to be accumulated in the belly, rather than on the hips and thighs.

While menopause is a fully normal part of the aging process, therapies such as estrogen therapy may lessen your risk of belly fat accumulation and its related health problems .

If you have concerns, contact with a healthcare practitioner or a registered dietitian nutritionist.

Natural hormonal changes during menopause result in a shift in fat storage from the hips and thighs to fat deposited around the belly.

7. The incorrect gut bacteria

Hundreds of species of bacteria exist in your gut, particularly in your colon. Some of these microorganisms enhance health, while others might create difficulties.

Gut bacteria are collectively known as your gut flora or microbiome. Gut health is vital for maintaining a healthy immune system and minimizing illness risk.

While the connection between the gut microbiome and health continues to be investigated, current research suggests imbalances in gut bacteria may increase your risk of developing a number of diseases, including type 2 diabetes, heart disease, obesity, and gut disorders (e.g., irritable bowel syndrome, inflammatory bowel disease) (e.g., irritable bowel syndrome, inflammatory bowel disease).

There's also some studies showing that having an improper mix of gut flora may promote weight growth, especially belly fat.

It's suspected that changes in bacteria variety may lead to alterations in energy and nutrition metabolism, promote inflammation, and disrupt hormone balance, leading to weight gain.

One randomized, double-blind 12-week research in postmenopausal women with obesity found that taking a probiotic comprising five strains of “good” bacteria led to substantial decreases in body fat percentage and visceral fat.

However, the limited sample size and uncontrolled diet caused difficulties .

While there seems to be a link between gut microbiome diversity and visceral obesity, additional study is required to fully understand its association and which therapies and probiotic strains may be most helpful.

Additionally, in general, consuming a low fiber diet heavy in sugar and saturated fat appears to be associated to harmful gut flora, while a fiber-dense diet rich in fruits and vegetables and whole, minimally processed foods seems to build a healthy gut.

Changes in bacteria diversity in the gut may be connected with greater weight and visceral fat.

8. Stress and cortisol

Cortisol is a hormone that's important for living.

It's generated by the adrenal glands and is known as a "stress hormone" because it helps your body react to a physical or psychological danger or stressor.

Today, most individuals experience chronic, low-grade stress rather than acute stress from an imminent danger (e.g., fleeing from a predator) (e.g., running from a predator).

The major stressors include psychological stress and actions that raise the likelihood of bad health outcomes (e.g., highly processed meals, physical inactivity, poor sleep) (e.g., highly processed diets, physical inactivity, poor sleep).

Unfortunately, persistent stress may contribute to the formation of visceral fat and making it hard to remove since it can boost production of cortisol in excess.

Furthermore, greater levels of cortisol in response to food may cause people to pick high-calorie meals for comfort, which may contribute to undesirable weight gain.

This may lead to overconsumption of meals heavy in fat and sugar, which are fast and dense types of energy, to prepare the body for the imagined danger. Nowadays with continuous stress, this meal is now eaten for comfort which may lead to overeating and ultimately weight gain.

Therefore, controlling your stress via health-promoting lifestyle choices (e.g., nutrient-dense diet, frequent exercise, meditation, treating mental health) and collaborating with a healthcare professional should be a focus.

The hormone cortisol, which is released in reaction to stress, may contribute to increased belly fat when in excess. Practicing healthy lifestyle practices is a vital component of managing chronic stress and keeping cortisol levels in control.

9. Low fiber diet

Fiber is highly essential for overall health and weight control.

Some forms of fiber may help you feel full, balance hunger hormones, and control appetite.

Diets heavy in refined carbohydrates and poor in fiber seem to have the opposite impact on hunger and weight gain, including increases in belly fat.

One big research including 2,854 people indicated that high-fiber whole grains were related with lower abdominal fat, whereas processed grains were connected to increased abdominal fat.

Foods rich in fiber include:

beans

lentils

entire grains

oats\svegetables\sfruit\splain popcorn

nuts seeds

A diet that's low in fiber and heavy in refined grains may raise risk for weight gain and greater levels of abdominal fat.

10. Genetics

Genes have a key impact in the risk of getting obese.

Similarly, it seems that the inclination to accumulate fat in the belly versus other areas of the body, is partially determined by heredity.

Interestingly, new research has begun to discover specific genes connected with obesity. For example, some genes may impact the secretion and activity of leptin, a hormone involved for hunger control and weight management.

While promising, much more study has to be undertaken in this area.

Though more study is required, genetics may have a role in where we store fat in the body, including higher risk for abdominal fat buildup.

11. Not enough sleep

Getting adequate sleep is vital for your health.

Many studies have connected insufficient sleep with weight growth, which may include belly fat.

There are numerous possible reasons of weight gain from lack of sleep, including increased food consumption to compensate for lack of energy, changes in hunger hormones, inflammation, and loss of physical activity owing to exhaustion.

For example, persons with insufficient sleep are more likely to pick low-nutrient alternatives (e.g., meals heavy in sugar and fat) and eat more calories daily than those who receive enough sleep each night.

What's more, sleep disturbances may also contribute to weight gain. One of the most frequent illnesses, sleep apnea, is a condition in which breathing pauses regularly throughout the night owing to soft tissue in the throat restricting the airway.

However, lack of sleep and weight growth offer a "chicken or the egg" problem. While sleep deprivation tends to contribute to weight growth, higher BMIs may lead to sleep difficulties and sleep disorders.

Short sleep or low-quality sleep may contribute to weight increase, particularly belly fat buildup.

Many distinct variables might increase the probability of accumulating extra belly fat.

There are a few things you can't do much about, such your genes and natural hormone changes after menopause. But there are also numerous aspects you do have the capacity to control.

Making health-promoting decisions about what to eat and what to avoid, how much you exercise, and how you manage stress may all help you shed belly fat and manage the related health risks.

Belly fat is the most dangerous fat in your body, connected to numerous ailments. Here are 6 easy techniques to reduce abdominal fat that are validated by research.

For a healthy diet, aim to consume more of these foods: vegetables, fruits, whole grains, lean proteins, and some low-fat dairy products.

Eating a nutritious diet and obtaining regular physical exercise are crucial ways to remain healthy and lower the possibility of acquiring numerous illnesses. In Kansas, nearly 35 percent of our population is overweight and almost one-third more is obese.

Having extra weight is a risk factor for several ailments, including coronary heart disease, stroke, Type 2 diabetes, osteoarthritis, sleep apnea, various malignancies, and more.

Start modestly by creating objectives that are more likely to be successful. Then gradually strive toward where you want to be. Setting realistic objectives will lead to permanent improvement.

Chapter 2

Here are 10 modest ways you may enhance your nutrition.

Keep your daily calorie consumption to a sensible quantity. Find out how many calories you need for your age, gender, exercise level, and weight objectives (i.e., do you want to lose, increase or maintain your weight?). To help calculate your calorie and nutritional requirements, If you wish to lose weight, see your health care practitioner for a safe calorie target and eating plan.

Working with other licensed advisors like a dietician, fitness professional, or wellness coach may assist and support you as you strive toward your objectives.

Enjoy your meal but eat less. Take time to savor what you are eating. This is called mindful eating. Eating hastily or without paying attention to what you eat, known as thoughtless ingesting, may lead to eating too many calories.

Keep portion amounts of meals to a fair and suggested level. To understand more about how much food to consume every day for your calorie requirements, in the fruits, vegetables, protein, and grains food categories, go to the super tracker website.

Try to consume more of these foods: vegetables, fruits, whole grains, lean proteins, and some low-fat dairy products. Try to make them the foundation for your meals and snacks rather than meats and other high-fat and non-nutritive items.

Dedicate half your plate at meals to fruits and vegetables. Fruits, vegetables (and grains) give vital vitamins, minerals, and phytochemicals. Most contain low fat and no cholesterol.

They also include fiber to aid with digestion and avoid constipation. Research reveals that eating a diet heavy in fruits and vegetables may help decrease cholesterol and blood sugar and avoid heart disease.

Try to make at least half (or ideally all) your daily grains whole grains. Foods prepared from whole grains are a primary source of energy and fiber. Learn to read food labels so you can discover which grains are genuinely whole grains.

Select leaner sources of protein and attempt to utilize more plant-based proteins in your meals and dishes. Protein foods include animal sources (meat, poultry, fish, eggs, and dairy products) and plant sources (beans, peas, soy products, nuts, seeds) (beans, peas, soy products, nuts, seeds).

Cut down on less healthful foods. These are foods heavy in saturated and solid (trans) fats and added sweets and salt, such as cookies, ice cream, candy, sweetened beverages, and fatty meats like bacon and hot dogs.

These meals often deliver a lot of calories and limited, if any, nutritional value. Have them as occasional treats but not every day.

Reduce your sodium (salt consumption) (salt intake). Cut down on consuming canned, packaged, and frozen processed foods.

If you are purchasing these things, utilize the Nutrition Facts label to find reduced salt versions of foods. High-sodium restaurant meals are also another key source of extra salt in one's diet.

Rethink your drink. Drink more water and other unsweetened liquids, instead of sugary and other high-calorie drinks. Soda, sweetened juice, energy, and sports drinks are key sources of added sugar and calories in many diets.

Chapter 3

The most effective exercises for losing weight

Plank posture for powerful legs, back, and abs

When many individuals think of reducing weight, one of the first things that come to mind is gaining a toned and taut belly. We hate to break it to you, but performing hundreds of crunches every day isn't the greatest method to reduce belly fat. In reality, workouts that promote spot reduction simply don't exist.

Burpees:This workout strengthens your core, as well as your chest, shoulders, lats, triceps, and quads. Since burpees entail intense plyometric action, they'll get your heart racing too.

How to perform burpees: Stand with your feet shoulder distance apart and send your hips back as you drop your body toward the ground in a low squat. Then, position your hands exactly outside of your feet and bounce your feet back, allowing your chest to contact the floor. Push your hands on the floor to elevate your body up into a plank and then hop your feet slightly outside of your hands. With your weight in your heels, spring explosively into the air with your arms aloft.

Mountain Climbers: How to do mountain climbers: Get into a high-plank stance with your wrists squarely beneath your shoulders. Keep your core firm, bringing your belly button in toward your spine. Drive your right knee toward your chest and then bring it back to plank. Then, push your left knee toward your chest and pull it back. Continue to alternate sides.

Turkish Get-Up The Turkish get-up is a 200-year-old total-body workout that requires utilizing a kettlebell, and it's a favorite of celebrity trainer Ramona Braganza. While it is a little complex, she believes that the total-body conditioning technique is truly beneficial.

How to perform a Turkish get-up: Holding one kettlebell by the grip with both hands, lay on your side in a fetal posture. Roll onto your back and push the kettlebell up toward the ceiling with both hands until the weight is steady on one loaded side. Release your free arm and a free leg to a 45-degree angle with your palm pointing down. Slide the heel of the weighted side closer to your butt to securely hold the floor.

Pushing through the foot on the floor, slam the kettlebell up with the laden arm and roll onto your free forearm. Don't shrug your shoulder toward your ear with the supporting side. Be careful to keep your chest wide open. Straighten the elbow on the ground and bring yourself up to a sitting posture. Weave your front leg across to the back. To protect your knees, your shin on the rear leg should be perpendicular to your shin on the front leg.

Perfectly line your arms: wrist over the elbow, shoulder over elbow over the wrist. Raise your torso to make your upper body erect. Swivel your back knee such that your back shin is parallel with your front shin. Get a hold on the floor with your back toes, then take a deep breath, and rise.

Medicine Ball Burpees

Phelps proposes adding a medicine ball to your burpee to improve the intensity of the workout and raise your metabolism—all while creating a sleek set of six-pack abs.

How to perform medicine ball burpees: Standing with your feet shoulder distance apart, grasp a medicine ball with both hands. Extend the ball up above, then smash the ball down on the ground as hard as you can, hinging over and seating your butt back as you slam. As you tilt over, bow your knees. Place your hands on the ground outside of your feet and bounce back into a high-plank stance. Keep your body in a straight line. Then, hop your feet back towards the outsides of your hands so that you are squatting. Pick up the ball and push it high, stretching your body and standing tall.

Sprawls push-ups:

The sprawl is simply a burpee on steroids—a complete body workout that works as many muscles as possible and burns calories while sculpting and toning your upper- and lower body, notably your abs. It takes the basic burpee to the next level by having you put your chest to the ground, then pushes up to plank while you continue the action.

How to perform a sprawl: Standing with your feet shoulder distance apart, crouch down, and put your hands on the ground. Jump your feet back to a plank and drop your body to contact the ground. Push yourself up to a plank and then hop your feet outside of your hands into a squat. Stand back up. That's one rep. If you want to burn even more calories, add a leap between each sprawl.

Side-to-Side Medicine Ball Slams:

Medicine ball slams are a dynamic, energetic, and highly metabolic workout that does not only target one muscle area. On the surface, the obliques, hamstrings, quadriceps, biceps, and shoulders are the key movers of this exercise. But as time goes on and weariness sets in, practically every other muscle in the body, in one way or another, may get engaged as a secondary action. Doing side-to-side ball smashes vs overhead slams combines greater oblique ab training.

How to execute lateral medicine ball slams: Stand with your feet approximately shoulder-width apart with the medicine ball on one side. Pick up the ball and just swivel your body while you smack the ball a few inches away from your pinky toe. Make careful to swivel your feet and bend the rear knee as you move into a split squat stance to grab the ball on one bounce. Alternate sides. Make sure you tense your core as you bring the ball above and to the side.

Overhead Medicine Ball Slams: Overhead medicine ball slams improve your core as it works against gravity. This workout also pushes your endurance, pushing your heart rate up each time you raise the ball and bring it above. You get the most out of this workout, make sure to utilize a hefty weighted ball.

Glycine ball with both hands. Reach both arms high, completely stretching your body. Slam the ball forward and down toward the ground. Extend your arms toward the ground as you smash and don't be scared to bend your knees as you tilt over. Squat to pick the ball up and then stand back up.

Russian Twists:\sThe Russian twist is a core workout that enhances oblique strength and definition.

The action, generally done with a medicine ball or plate, includes twisting your torso from side to side while keeping a sit-up posture with your feet off the ground.

How to perform Russian twists: Sit up straight on the floor with your knees bent and feet off the ground. Hold a medicine ball with your hands at chest height.

Lean backward with a long, tall spine, holding your body at a 45-degree angle and maintaining your arms a few inches apart from your chest.

From here, turn your body to the right, stop and squeeze your right oblique muscles, then shift your torso to the left and pause to tighten your left oblique muscles. The movement should originate from your ribcage and not your arm.

BOSU Ball Planks:

You know that your cardio exercises are vital when it comes to burning the layer of fat lying on top of your abdominal muscles. But it's still crucial to train those abs even when you're attempting to lose weight.

It's more demanding than a typical plank when your hands are on the floor since the BOSU challenges your balance.

When your body strives to establish control when your balance is tested, your abs, obliques, and deep transverse abdominal muscles are recruited. Strengthening these core muscles also helps raise your metabolism, eventually allowing you to burn more calories and fat.

How to perform BOSU ball planks: Flip a BOSU ball on its rubber side and grab onto the sides of the flat surface with both hands, roughly shoulder distance apart.

Hold the plank for 30 to 45 seconds, increasing the duration as you grow stronger.

Jogging On an Incline:

Running at an inclination rather than on a level surface has been demonstrated to enhance overall calorie burn by as much as 50 percent.

Whether you're outdoors on a hill or in the gym on an inclined treadmill, start off walking for five to 10 minutes. Your heart rate should climb quite fast as you ramp up your speed.

Try this treadmill workout: Walk or jog on an incline for five to 10 minutes. Maintain a jog for another five to 10 minutes, then push your speed up again and start running.

This doesn't have to be an all-out sprint, but you should be working hard enough that you can't have a conversation. Spend five minutes running, then reduce your speed back down to a jog.

Continue alternating with five to 10 minutes of jogging and five to 10 minutes of running for 30 to 45 minutes.

www.ingramcontent.com/pod-product-compliance
Lightning Source LLC
LaVergne TN
LVHW050348160826
845677LV00014B/3860
9798845698995